Today's Goal _______________   Ⓜ Ⓣ Ⓦ Ⓣ Ⓕ ⬤ ⬤

Muscle Group Focus _______________ Weight_________ Date/Time_________

Stretch ◯   Warm-Up _______________________________________

Strength Training

Exercise		Set 1	Set 2	Set 3	Set 4	Set 5	Set 6
	Reps						
	Weight						
	Reps						
	Weight						
	Reps						
	Weight						
	Reps						
	Weight						
	Reps						
	Weight						
	Reps						
	Weight						
	Reps						
	Weight						
	Reps						
	Weight						
	Reps						
	Weight						

Cardio

Exercise	Calories	Distance	Time

Water Intake _______________

Cooldown _______________

Feeling ☆ ☆ ☆ ☆ ☆

Notes

Today's Goal _______________   Ⓜ Ⓣ Ⓦ Ⓣ Ⓕ Ⓢ Ⓢ

Muscle Group Focus _______________ Weight________ Date/Time ________

Stretch ◯   Warm-Up _______________________________________

Strength Training

Exercise		Set 1	Set 2	Set 3	Set 4	Set 5	Set 6
	Reps						
	Weight						
	Reps						
	Weight						
	Reps						
	Weight						
	Reps						
	Weight						
	Reps						
	Weight						
	Reps						
	Weight						
	Reps						
	Weight						
	Reps						
	Weight						
	Reps						
	Weight						

Cardio

Exercise	Calories	Distance	Time

Water Intake _______________

Cooldown _______________

Feeling ☆ ☆ ☆ ☆ ☆

Notes

Today's Goal _______________   Ⓜ Ⓣ Ⓦ Ⓣ Ⓕ **S** **S**

Muscle Group Focus _______________ Weight_________   Date/Time_________

Stretch ◯   Warm-Up ____

Strength Training

Exercise		Set 1	Set 2	Set 3	Set 4	Set 5	Set 6
	Reps						
	Weight						
	Reps						
	Weight						
	Reps						
	Weight						
	Reps						
	Weight						
	Reps						
	Weight						
	Reps						
	Weight						
	Reps						
	Weight						
	Reps						
	Weight						
	Reps						
	Weight						
	Reps						
	Weight						

Cardio

Exercise	Calories	Distance	Time

Water Intake _______________

Cooldown _______________

Feeling ☆ ☆ ☆ ☆ ☆

Notes

Today's Goal ______________   (M) (T) (W) (T) (F) **(S)** **(S)**

Muscle Group Focus _____________ Weight_______ Date/Time _______

Stretch ◯   Warm-Up _______________________________

Strength Training

Exercise		Set 1	Set 2	Set 3	Set 4	Set 5	Set 6
	Reps						
	Weight						
	Reps						
	Weight						
	Reps						
	Weight						
	Reps						
	Weight						
	Reps						
	Weight						
	Reps						
	Weight						
	Reps						
	Weight						
	Reps						
	Weight						
	Reps						
	Weight						
	Reps						
	Weight						

Cardio

Exercise	Calories	Distance	Time

Water Intake _______________

Cooldown ______________

Feeling ☆ ☆ ☆ ☆ ☆

Notes

Today's Goal   _______________   (M) (T) (W) (T) (F) (S) (S)

Muscle Group Focus   _____________ Weight_________   Date/Time _________

Stretch ◯   Warm-Up ____

Strength Training

Exercise		Set 1	Set 2	Set 3	Set 4	Set 5	Set 6
	Reps						
	Weight						
	Reps						
	Weight						
	Reps						
	Weight						
	Reps						
	Weight						
	Reps						
	Weight						
	Reps						
	Weight						
	Reps						
	Weight						
	Reps						
	Weight						
	Reps						
	Weight						
	Reps						
	Weight						

Cardio

Exercise	Calories	Distance	Time

Water Intake _______________

Cooldown _______________

Feeling ☆ ☆ ☆ ☆ ☆

Notes

Today's Goal ______________ (M) (T) (W) (T) (F) (S) (S)

Muscle Group Focus ____________ Weight________ Date/Time ________

Stretch ◯   Warm–Up __________________________________

Strength Training

Exercise		Set 1	Set 2	Set 3	Set 4	Set 5	Set 6
	Reps						
	Weight						
	Reps						
	Weight						
	Reps						
	Weight						
	Reps						
	Weight						
	Reps						
	Weight						
	Reps						
	Weight						
	Reps						
	Weight						
	Reps						
	Weight						
	Reps						
	Weight						
	Reps						
	Weight						

Cardio

Exercise	Calories	Distance	Time

Water Intake _______________

Cooldown _______________

Feeling ☆ ☆ ☆ ☆ ☆

Notes

Today's Goal _______________   (M) (T) (W) (T) (F) (S) (S)

Muscle Group Focus _______________ Weight_________ Date/Time _______

Stretch ○   Warm-Up ____

Strength Training

Exercise		Set 1	Set 2	Set 3	Set 4	Set 5	Set 6
	Reps						
	Weight						
	Reps						
	Weight						
	Reps						
	Weight						
	Reps						
	Weight						
	Reps						
	Weight						
	Reps						
	Weight						
	Reps						
	Weight						
	Reps						
	Weight						
	Reps						
	Weight						
	Reps						
	Weight						

Cardio

Exercise	Calories	Distance	Time

Water Intake _________________

Cooldown _________________

Feeling ☆ ☆ ☆ ☆ ☆

Notes

Today's Goal _______________ Ⓜ Ⓣ Ⓦ Ⓣ Ⓕ Ⓢ Ⓢ

Muscle Group Focus _______________ Weight________ Date/Time ________

Stretch ◯   Warm-Up ____

Strength Training

Exercise		Set 1	Set 2	Set 3	Set 4	Set 5	Set 6
	Reps						
	Weight						
	Reps						
	Weight						
	Reps						
	Weight						
	Reps						
	Weight						
	Reps						
	Weight						
	Reps						
	Weight						
	Reps						
	Weight						
	Reps						
	Weight						
	Reps						
	Weight						
	Reps						
	Weight						

Cardio

Exercise	Calories	Distance	Time

Water Intake ___________________

Cooldown ___________________

Feeling ☆ ☆ ☆ ☆ ☆

Notes

Today's Goal _______________

(M) (T) (W) (T) (F) (S) (S)

Muscle Group Focus _____________ Weight_______ Date/Time_______

Stretch ◯   Warm-Up _______________________________

Strength Training

Exercise		Set 1	Set 2	Set 3	Set 4	Set 5	Set 6
	Reps						
	Weight						
	Reps						
	Weight						
	Reps						
	Weight						
	Reps						
	Weight						
	Reps						
	Weight						
	Reps						
	Weight						
	Reps						
	Weight						
	Reps						
	Weight						
	Reps						
	Weight						

Cardio

Exercise	Calories	Distance	Time

Water Intake ________________

Cooldown _______________

Feeling ☆ ☆ ☆ ☆ ☆

Notes

Today's Goal ______________   Ⓜ Ⓣ Ⓦ Ⓣ Ⓕ **Ⓢ** **Ⓢ**

Muscle Group Focus ______________ Weight________   Date/Time________

Stretch ◯   Warm-Up ____________________________

Strength Training

Exercise		Set 1	Set 2	Set 3	Set 4	Set 5	Set 6
	Reps						
	Weight						
	Reps						
	Weight						
	Reps						
	Weight						
	Reps						
	Weight						
	Reps						
	Weight						
	Reps						
	Weight						
	Reps						
	Weight						
	Reps						
	Weight						
	Reps						
	Weight						
	Reps						
	Weight						

Cardio

Exercise	Calories	Distance	Time

Water Intake ______________

Cooldown ______________

Feeling ☆ ☆ ☆ ☆ ☆

Notes

Today's Goal _______________ (M) (T) (W) (T) (F) (S) (S)

Muscle Group Focus _______________ Weight_________ Date/Time_________

Stretch ◯   Warm-Up _______________________________________

Strength Training

Exercise		Set 1	Set 2	Set 3	Set 4	Set 5	Set 6
	Reps						
	Weight						
	Reps						
	Weight						
	Reps						
	Weight						
	Reps						
	Weight						
	Reps						
	Weight						
	Reps						
	Weight						
	Reps						
	Weight						
	Reps						
	Weight						
	Reps						
	Weight						

Cardio

Exercise	Calories	Distance	Time

Water Intake _______________

Cooldown _______________

Feeling ☆ ☆ ☆ ☆ ☆

Notes

Today's Goal   _________________   (M) (T) (W) (T) (F) (S) (S)

Muscle Group Focus _______________ Weight_________   Date/Time ________

Stretch ◯   Warm-Up ____________________________________

Strength Training

Exercise		Set 1	Set 2	Set 3	Set 4	Set 5	Set 6
	Reps						
	Weight						
	Reps						
	Weight						
	Reps						
	Weight						
	Reps						
	Weight						
	Reps						
	Weight						
	Reps						
	Weight						
	Reps						
	Weight						
	Reps						
	Weight						
	Reps						
	Weight						
	Reps						
	Weight						

Cardio

Exercise	Calories	Distance	Time

Water Intake _________________

Cooldown _________________

Feeling ☆ ☆ ☆ ☆ ☆

Notes

Today's Goal _______________ Ⓜ Ⓣ Ⓦ Ⓣ Ⓕ Ⓢ Ⓢ

Muscle Group Focus _____________ Weight________ Date/Time________

Stretch ◯   Warm-Up _________________________________

Strength Training

Exercise		Set 1	Set 2	Set 3	Set 4	Set 5	Set 6
	Reps						
	Weight						
	Reps						
	Weight						
	Reps						
	Weight						
	Reps						
	Weight						
	Reps						
	Weight						
	Reps						
	Weight						
	Reps						
	Weight						
	Reps						
	Weight						
	Reps						
	Weight						

Cardio

Exercise	Calories	Distance	Time

Water Intake _________________

Cooldown _______________

Feeling ☆ ☆ ☆ ☆ ☆

Notes

Today's Goal ______________   (M) (T) (W) (T) (F) (S) (S)

Muscle Group Focus ______________ Weight________   Date/Time________

Stretch ◯   Warm-Up ________________________________

Strength Training

Exercise		Set 1	Set 2	Set 3	Set 4	Set 5	Set 6
	Reps						
	Weight						
	Reps						
	Weight						
	Reps						
	Weight						
	Reps						
	Weight						
	Reps						
	Weight						
	Reps						
	Weight						
	Reps						
	Weight						
	Reps						
	Weight						
	Reps						
	Weight						
	Reps						
	Weight						

Cardio

Exercise	Calories	Distance	Time

Water Intake ______________

Cooldown ______________

Feeling ☆ ☆ ☆ ☆ ☆

Notes

Today's Goal _______________   (M) (T) (W) (T) (F) (S) (S)

Muscle Group Focus _______________ Weight________   Date/Time________

Stretch ◯   Warm-Up ____

Strength Training

Exercise		Set 1	Set 2	Set 3	Set 4	Set 5	Set 6
	Reps						
	Weight						
	Reps						
	Weight						
	Reps						
	Weight						
	Reps						
	Weight						
	Reps						
	Weight						
	Reps						
	Weight						
	Reps						
	Weight						
	Reps						
	Weight						
	Reps						
	Weight						

Cardio

Exercise	Calories	Distance	Time

Water Intake _______________

Cooldown _______________

Feeling ☆ ☆ ☆ ☆ ☆

Notes

Today's Goal _______________   (M) (T) (W) (T) (F) (S) (S)

Muscle Group Focus _______________ Weight_________   Date/Time_________

Stretch ◯   Warm-Up _________________________________

Strength Training

Exercise			Set 1	Set 2	Set 3	Set 4	Set 5	Set 6
		Reps						
		Weight						
		Reps						
		Weight						
		Reps						
		Weight						
		Reps						
		Weight						
		Reps						
		Weight						
		Reps						
		Weight						
		Reps						
		Weight						
		Reps						
		Weight						
		Reps						
		Weight						
		Reps						
		Weight						

Cardio

Exercise	Calories	Distance	Time

Water Intake _________________

Cooldown _________________

Feeling ☆ ☆ ☆ ☆ ☆

Notes

Today's Goal _______________ Ⓜ Ⓣ Ⓦ Ⓣ Ⓕ ⚫S ⚫S

Muscle Group Focus _______________ Weight_________ Date/Time ________

Stretch ◯   Warm-Up ____

Strength Training

Exercise		Set 1	Set 2	Set 3	Set 4	Set 5	Set 6
	Reps						
	Weight						
	Reps						
	Weight						
	Reps						
	Weight						
	Reps						
	Weight						
	Reps						
	Weight						
	Reps						
	Weight						
	Reps						
	Weight						
	Reps						
	Weight						
	Reps						
	Weight						
	Reps						
	Weight						

Cardio

Exercise	Calories	Distance	Time

Water Intake _______________

Cooldown _______________

Feeling ☆ ☆ ☆ ☆ ☆

Notes

Today's Goal _______________   Ⓜ Ⓣ Ⓦ Ⓣ Ⓕ ⬤S ⬤S

Muscle Group Focus _______________ Weight________ Date/Time________

Stretch ◯   Warm-Up ______________________________

Strength Training

Exercise		Set 1	Set 2	Set 3	Set 4	Set 5	Set 6
	Reps						
	Weight						
	Reps						
	Weight						
	Reps						
	Weight						
	Reps						
	Weight						
	Reps						
	Weight						
	Reps						
	Weight						
	Reps						
	Weight						
	Reps						
	Weight						
	Reps						
	Weight						
	Reps						
	Weight						

Cardio

Exercise	Calories	Distance	Time

Water Intake _______________

Cooldown _______________

Feeling ☆ ☆ ☆ ☆ ☆

Notes

Today's Goal _______________ (M) (T) (W) (T) (F) (S) (S)

Muscle Group Focus _______________ Weight_________ Date/Time_________

Stretch ○   Warm-Up _______________________________________

Strength Training

Exercise		Set 1	Set 2	Set 3	Set 4	Set 5	Set 6
	Reps						
	Weight						
	Reps						
	Weight						
	Reps						
	Weight						
	Reps						
	Weight						
	Reps						
	Weight						
	Reps						
	Weight						
	Reps						
	Weight						
	Reps						
	Weight						
	Reps						
	Weight						
	Reps						
	Weight						

Cardio

Exercise	Calories	Distance	Time

Water Intake _______________

Cooldown _______________

Feeling ☆ ☆ ☆ ☆ ☆

Notes

Today's Goal ________________

(M) (T) (W) (T) (F) (S) (S)

Muscle Group Focus ______________Weight________ Date/Time_______

Stretch ◯   Warm-Up _________________________________

Strength Training

Exercise		Set 1	Set 2	Set 3	Set 4	Set 5	Set 6
	Reps						
	Weight						
	Reps						
	Weight						
	Reps						
	Weight						
	Reps						
	Weight						
	Reps						
	Weight						
	Reps						
	Weight						
	Reps						
	Weight						
	Reps						
	Weight						
	Reps						
	Weight						
	Reps						
	Weight						

Cardio

Exercise	Calories	Distance	Time

Water Intake ______________

Cooldown ______________

Feeling ☆ ☆ ☆ ☆ ☆

Notes

Today's Goal ___________ (M) (T) (W) (T) (F) (S) (S)

Muscle Group Focus ___________ Weight_______ Date/Time_______

Stretch ◯   Warm-Up ______________________________

Strength Training

Exercise		Set 1	Set 2	Set 3	Set 4	Set 5	Set 6
	Reps						
	Weight						
	Reps						
	Weight						
	Reps						
	Weight						
	Reps						
	Weight						
	Reps						
	Weight						
	Reps						
	Weight						
	Reps						
	Weight						
	Reps						
	Weight						
	Reps						
	Weight						
	Reps						
	Weight						

Cardio

Exercise	Calories	Distance	Time

Water Intake ______________

Cooldown _____________

Feeling ☆ ☆ ☆ ☆ ☆

Notes

Today's Goal ___________________

(M) (T) (W) (T) (F) (S) (S)

Muscle Group Focus _______________Weight_________   Date/Time________

Stretch ◯   Warm-Up ____

Strength Training

Exercise		Set 1	Set 2	Set 3	Set 4	Set 5	Set 6
	Reps						
	Weight						
	Reps						
	Weight						
	Reps						
	Weight						
	Reps						
	Weight						
	Reps						
	Weight						
	Reps						
	Weight						
	Reps						
	Weight						
	Reps						
	Weight						
	Reps						
	Weight						
	Reps						
	Weight						

Cardio

Exercise	Calories	Distance	Time

Water Intake ___________________

Cooldown ___________________

Feeling ☆ ☆ ☆ ☆ ☆

Notes

Today's Goal _______________ (M) (T) (W) (T) (F) (S) (S)

Muscle Group Focus _______________ Weight________ Date/Time ________

Stretch ◯   **Warm-Up** _______________________________________

Strength Training

Exercise		Set 1	Set 2	Set 3	Set 4	Set 5	Set 6
	Reps						
	Weight						
	Reps						
	Weight						
	Reps						
	Weight						
	Reps						
	Weight						
	Reps						
	Weight						
	Reps						
	Weight						
	Reps						
	Weight						
	Reps						
	Weight						
	Reps						
	Weight						
	Reps						
	Weight						

Cardio

Exercise	Calories	Distance	Time

Water Intake _______________

Cooldown _______________

Feeling ☆ ☆ ☆ ☆ ☆

Notes

Today's Goal _______________   (M) (T) (W) (T) (F) (S) (S)

Muscle Group Focus _______________ Weight_________   Date/Time _________

Stretch ◯   Warm-Up _______________________________________

Strength Training

Exercise		Set 1	Set 2	Set 3	Set 4	Set 5	Set 6
	Reps						
	Weight						
	Reps						
	Weight						
	Reps						
	Weight						
	Reps						
	Weight						
	Reps						
	Weight						
	Reps						
	Weight						
	Reps						
	Weight						
	Reps						
	Weight						
	Reps						
	Weight						
	Reps						
	Weight						

Cardio

Exercise	Calories	Distance	Time

Water Intake _______________

Cooldown _______________

Feeling ☆ ☆ ☆ ☆ ☆

Notes

Today's Goal ________________ (M) (T) (W) (T) (F) (S) (S)

Muscle Group Focus ______________ Weight_________ Date/Time________

Stretch ◯   Warm-Up ____________________________________

Strength Training

Exercise		Set 1	Set 2	Set 3	Set 4	Set 5	Set 6
	Reps						
	Weight						
	Reps						
	Weight						
	Reps						
	Weight						
	Reps						
	Weight						
	Reps						
	Weight						
	Reps						
	Weight						
	Reps						
	Weight						
	Reps						
	Weight						
	Reps						
	Weight						
	Reps						
	Weight						

Cardio

Exercise	Calories	Distance	Time

Water Intake _________________

Cooldown ______________

Feeling ☆ ☆ ☆ ☆ ☆

Notes

Today's Goal _______________

M T W T F **S** **S**

Muscle Group Focus _______________ Weight_________ Date/Time _______

Stretch ◯ Warm-Up ____

Strength Training

Exercise		Set 1	Set 2	Set 3	Set 4	Set 5	Set 6
	Reps						
	Weight						
	Reps						
	Weight						
	Reps						
	Weight						
	Reps						
	Weight						
	Reps						
	Weight						
	Reps						
	Weight						
	Reps						
	Weight						
	Reps						
	Weight						
	Reps						
	Weight						
	Reps						
	Weight						

Cardio

Exercise	Calories	Distance	Time

Water Intake _______________

Cooldown _______________

Feeling ☆ ☆ ☆ ☆ ☆

Notes

Today's Goal _____________

(M) (T) (W) (T) (F) **S** **S**

Muscle Group Focus ____________Weight_______ Date/Time_______

Stretch ◯ Warm-Up __________________________

Strength Training

Exercise		Set 1	Set 2	Set 3	Set 4	Set 5	Set 6
	Reps						
	Weight						
	Reps						
	Weight						
	Reps						
	Weight						
	Reps						
	Weight						
	Reps						
	Weight						
	Reps						
	Weight						
	Reps						
	Weight						
	Reps						
	Weight						
	Reps						
	Weight						

Cardio

Exercise	Calories	Distance	Time

Water Intake _______________

Cooldown _____________

Feeling ☆ ☆ ☆ ☆ ☆

Notes

Today's Goal _______________

(M) (T) (W) (T) (F) **S** **S**

Muscle Group Focus _____________Weight________ Date/Time ________

Stretch ◯ Warm-Up _________________________________

Strength Training

Exercise		Set 1	Set 2	Set 3	Set 4	Set 5	Set 6
	Reps						
	Weight						
	Reps						
	Weight						
	Reps						
	Weight						
	Reps						
	Weight						
	Reps						
	Weight						
	Reps						
	Weight						
	Reps						
	Weight						
	Reps						
	Weight						
	Reps						
	Weight						
	Reps						
	Weight						

Cardio

Exercise	Calories	Distance	Time

Water Intake _______________

Cooldown ______________

Feeling ☆ ☆ ☆ ☆ ☆

Notes

Today's Goal _______________

(M) (T) (W) (T) (F) (S) (S)

Muscle Group Focus ____________ Weight_______ Date/Time_______

Stretch ◯   Warm-Up _________________________________

Strength Training

Exercise		Set 1	Set 2	Set 3	Set 4	Set 5	Set 6
	Reps						
	Weight						
	Reps						
	Weight						
	Reps						
	Weight						
	Reps						
	Weight						
	Reps						
	Weight						
	Reps						
	Weight						
	Reps						
	Weight						
	Reps						
	Weight						
	Reps						
	Weight						
	Reps						
	Weight						

Cardio

Exercise	Calories	Distance	Time

Water Intake ______________

Cooldown ______________

Feeling ☆☆☆☆☆

Notes

Today's Goal ______________________________   (M) (T) (W) (T) (F) (S) (S)

Muscle Group Focus _________________ Weight_________ Date/Time _________

Stretch ◯   Warm-Up ____

Strength Training

Exercise		Set 1	Set 2	Set 3	Set 4	Set 5	Set 6
	Reps						
	Weight						
	Reps						
	Weight						
	Reps						
	Weight						
	Reps						
	Weight						
	Reps						
	Weight						
	Reps						
	Weight						
	Reps						
	Weight						
	Reps						
	Weight						
	Reps						
	Weight						
	Reps						
	Weight						

Cardio

Exercise	Calories	Distance	Time

Water Intake ____________________

Cooldown ____________________

Feeling ☆ ☆ ☆ ☆ ☆

Notes

Today's Goal ______________   (M) (T) (W) (T) (F) (S) (S)

Muscle Group Focus _____________ Weight________   Date/Time ________

Stretch ◯   Warm-Up ___________________________________

Strength Training

Exercise		Set 1	Set 2	Set 3	Set 4	Set 5	Set 6
	Reps						
	Weight						
	Reps						
	Weight						
	Reps						
	Weight						
	Reps						
	Weight						
	Reps						
	Weight						
	Reps						
	Weight						
	Reps						
	Weight						
	Reps						
	Weight						
	Reps						
	Weight						

Cardio

Exercise	Calories	Distance	Time

Water Intake ________________

Cooldown _______________

Feeling ☆ ☆ ☆ ☆ ☆

Notes

Today's Goal _____________   (M) (T) (W) (T) (F) (S) (S)

Muscle Group Focus ___________Weight_______   Date/Time_______

Stretch ◯   Warm-Up ______________________________________

Strength Training

Exercise		Set 1	Set 2	Set 3	Set 4	Set 5	Set 6
	Reps						
	Weight						
	Reps						
	Weight						
	Reps						
	Weight						
	Reps						
	Weight						
	Reps						
	Weight						
	Reps						
	Weight						
	Reps						
	Weight						
	Reps						
	Weight						
	Reps						
	Weight						
	Reps						
	Weight						

Cardio

Exercise	Calories	Distance	Time

Water Intake ________________

Cooldown _____________

Feeling ☆ ☆ ☆ ☆ ☆

Notes

Today's Goal _______________ Ⓜ Ⓣ Ⓦ Ⓣ Ⓕ ⬤S ⬤S

Muscle Group Focus _____________ Weight________ Date/Time ________

Stretch ◯   **Warm-Up** _______________________________

Strength Training

Exercise		Set 1	Set 2	Set 3	Set 4	Set 5	Set 6
	Reps						
	Weight						
	Reps						
	Weight						
	Reps						
	Weight						
	Reps						
	Weight						
	Reps						
	Weight						
	Reps						
	Weight						
	Reps						
	Weight						
	Reps						
	Weight						
	Reps						
	Weight						

Cardio

Exercise	Calories	Distance	Time

Water Intake _______________

Cooldown _______________

Feeling ☆ ☆ ☆ ☆ ☆

Notes

Today's Goal _________________ Ⓜ Ⓣ Ⓦ Ⓣ Ⓕ ⬤S ⬤S

Muscle Group Focus _______________ Weight_________ Date/Time_________

Stretch ◯   Warm-Up ____

Strength Training

Exercise		Set 1	Set 2	Set 3	Set 4	Set 5	Set 6
	Reps						
	Weight						
	Reps						
	Weight						
	Reps						
	Weight						
	Reps						
	Weight						
	Reps						
	Weight						
	Reps						
	Weight						
	Reps						
	Weight						
	Reps						
	Weight						
	Reps						
	Weight						
	Reps						
	Weight						

Cardio

Exercise	Calories	Distance	Time

Water Intake _______________

Cooldown _______________

Feeling ☆ ☆ ☆ ☆ ☆

Notes

Today's Goal   ____________   (M) (T) (W) (T) (F) (S) (S)

Muscle Group Focus ____________ Weight________ Date/Time _______

Stretch ◯   Warm-Up _________________________________

Strength Training

Exercise		Set 1	Set 2	Set 3	Set 4	Set 5	Set 6
	Reps						
	Weight						
	Reps						
	Weight						
	Reps						
	Weight						
	Reps						
	Weight						
	Reps						
	Weight						
	Reps						
	Weight						
	Reps						
	Weight						
	Reps						
	Weight						
	Reps						
	Weight						
	Reps						
	Weight						

Cardio

Exercise	Calories	Distance	Time

Water Intake _________________

Cooldown _________________

Feeling ☆ ☆ ☆ ☆ ☆

Notes

Today's Goal _______________

(M) (T) (W) (T) (F) **S** **S**

Muscle Group Focus _______________ Weight________ Date/Time _________

Stretch ○   Warm-Up _________________________________

Strength Training

Exercise		Set 1	Set 2	Set 3	Set 4	Set 5	Set 6
	Reps						
	Weight						
	Reps						
	Weight						
	Reps						
	Weight						
	Reps						
	Weight						
	Reps						
	Weight						
	Reps						
	Weight						
	Reps						
	Weight						
	Reps						
	Weight						
	Reps						
	Weight						
	Reps						
	Weight						

Cardio

Exercise	Calories	Distance	Time

Water Intake _______________

Cooldown _______________

Feeling ☆ ☆ ☆ ☆ ☆

Notes

Today's Goal _______________   Ⓜ Ⓣ Ⓦ Ⓣ Ⓕ ● ●

Muscle Group Focus _______________ Weight________ Date/Time________

Stretch ◯   Warm-Up _________________________________

Strength Training

Exercise		Set 1	Set 2	Set 3	Set 4	Set 5	Set 6
	Reps						
	Weight						
	Reps						
	Weight						
	Reps						
	Weight						
	Reps						
	Weight						
	Reps						
	Weight						
	Reps						
	Weight						
	Reps						
	Weight						
	Reps						
	Weight						
	Reps						
	Weight						
	Reps						
	Weight						

Cardio

Exercise	Calories	Distance	Time

Water Intake _______________

Cooldown _______________

Feeling ☆ ☆ ☆ ☆ ☆

Notes

Today's Goal _________________ Ⓜ Ⓣ Ⓦ Ⓣ Ⓕ ⚫ ⚫

Muscle Group Focus _____________ Weight_______ Date/Time_______

Stretch ◯   Warm-Up ____

Strength Training

Exercise		Set 1	Set 2	Set 3	Set 4	Set 5	Set 6
	Reps						
	Weight						
	Reps						
	Weight						
	Reps						
	Weight						
	Reps						
	Weight						
	Reps						
	Weight						
	Reps						
	Weight						
	Reps						
	Weight						
	Reps						
	Weight						
	Reps						
	Weight						
	Reps						
	Weight						

Cardio

Exercise	Calories	Distance	Time

Water Intake _________________

Cooldown _________________

Feeling ☆ ☆ ☆ ☆ ☆

Notes

Today's Goal _______________   (M) (T) (W) (T) (F) (S) (S)

Muscle Group Focus _______________ Weight_________   Date/Time_________

Stretch ◯   Warm-Up ____

Strength Training

Exercise		Set 1	Set 2	Set 3	Set 4	Set 5	Set 6
	Reps						
	Weight						
	Reps						
	Weight						
	Reps						
	Weight						
	Reps						
	Weight						
	Reps						
	Weight						
	Reps						
	Weight						
	Reps						
	Weight						
	Reps						
	Weight						
	Reps						
	Weight						

Cardio

Exercise	Calories	Distance	Time

Water Intake _______________

Cooldown _______________

Feeling ☆ ☆ ☆ ☆ ☆

Notes

Today's Goal ______________

(M) (T) (W) (T) (F) (S) (S)

Muscle Group Focus ____________ Weight________ Date/Time________

Stretch ◯   Warm-Up ____________________________________

Strength Training

Exercise		Set 1	Set 2	Set 3	Set 4	Set 5	Set 6
	Reps						
	Weight						
	Reps						
	Weight						
	Reps						
	Weight						
	Reps						
	Weight						
	Reps						
	Weight						
	Reps						
	Weight						
	Reps						
	Weight						
	Reps						
	Weight						
	Reps						
	Weight						
	Reps						
	Weight						

Cardio

Exercise	Calories	Distance	Time

Water Intake ______________

Cooldown ______________

Feeling ☆ ☆ ☆ ☆ ☆

Notes

Today's Goal _______________   Ⓜ Ⓣ Ⓦ Ⓣ Ⓕ **S** **S**

Muscle Group Focus _______________ Weight_________   Date/Time _________

Stretch ◯   Warm-Up _______________________________________

Strength Training

Exercise		Set 1	Set 2	Set 3	Set 4	Set 5	Set 6
	Reps						
	Weight						
	Reps						
	Weight						
	Reps						
	Weight						
	Reps						
	Weight						
	Reps						
	Weight						
	Reps						
	Weight						
	Reps						
	Weight						
	Reps						
	Weight						
	Reps						
	Weight						
	Reps						
	Weight						

Cardio

Exercise	Calories	Distance	Time

Water Intake _______________

Cooldown _______________

Feeling ☆ ☆ ☆ ☆ ☆

Notes

Today's Goal _______________   (M) (T) (W) (T) (F) **S** **S**

Muscle Group Focus _______________ Weight_________   Date/Time_________

Stretch ◯   Warm-Up _________________________________

Strength Training

Exercise			Set 1	Set 2	Set 3	Set 4	Set 5	Set 6
		Reps						
		Weight						
		Reps						
		Weight						
		Reps						
		Weight						
		Reps						
		Weight						
		Reps						
		Weight						
		Reps						
		Weight						
		Reps						
		Weight						
		Reps						
		Weight						
		Reps						
		Weight						
		Reps						
		Weight						

Cardio

Exercise	Calories	Distance	Time

Water Intake _______________

Cooldown _______________

Feeling ☆ ☆ ☆ ☆ ☆

Notes

Today's Goal _______________ (M) (T) (W) (T) (F) (S) (S)

Muscle Group Focus _______________ Weight_________ Date/Time_________

Stretch ◯   Warm-Up ____

Strength Training

Exercise		Set 1	Set 2	Set 3	Set 4	Set 5	Set 6
	Reps						
	Weight						
	Reps						
	Weight						
	Reps						
	Weight						
	Reps						
	Weight						
	Reps						
	Weight						
	Reps						
	Weight						
	Reps						
	Weight						
	Reps						
	Weight						
	Reps						
	Weight						
	Reps						
	Weight						

Cardio

Exercise	Calories	Distance	Time

Water Intake _______________

Cooldown _______________

Feeling ☆ ☆ ☆ ☆ ☆

Notes

Today's Goal __________________   Ⓜ Ⓣ Ⓦ Ⓣ Ⓕ ⬤S ⬤S

Muscle Group Focus __________________Weight_________   Date/Time_______

Stretch ◯   Warm-Up ____

Strength Training

Exercise		Set 1	Set 2	Set 3	Set 4	Set 5	Set 6
	Reps						
	Weight						
	Reps						
	Weight						
	Reps						
	Weight						
	Reps						
	Weight						
	Reps						
	Weight						
	Reps						
	Weight						
	Reps						
	Weight						
	Reps						
	Weight						
	Reps						
	Weight						
	Reps						
	Weight						

Cardio

Exercise	Calories	Distance	Time

Water Intake __________________

Cooldown __________________

Feeling ☆ ☆ ☆ ☆ ☆

Notes

Today's Goal _________________ Ⓜ Ⓣ Ⓦ Ⓣ Ⓕ ⬤S ⬤S

Muscle Group Focus _____________ Weight________ Date/Time_______

Stretch ◯   Warm-Up ________________________________

Strength Training

Exercise		Set 1	Set 2	Set 3	Set 4	Set 5	Set 6
	Reps						
	Weight						
	Reps						
	Weight						
	Reps						
	Weight						
	Reps						
	Weight						
	Reps						
	Weight						
	Reps						
	Weight						
	Reps						
	Weight						
	Reps						
	Weight						
	Reps						
	Weight						

Cardio

Exercise	Calories	Distance	Time

Water Intake _______________

Cooldown _______________

Feeling ☆ ☆ ☆ ☆ ☆

Notes

Today's Goal _______________

(M) (T) (W) (T) (F) (S) (S)

Muscle Group Focus _______________ Weight_________ Date/Time_________

Stretch ◯   Warm-Up _______________________________________

Strength Training

Exercise		Set 1	Set 2	Set 3	Set 4	Set 5	Set 6
	Reps						
	Weight						
	Reps						
	Weight						
	Reps						
	Weight						
	Reps						
	Weight						
	Reps						
	Weight						
	Reps						
	Weight						
	Reps						
	Weight						
	Reps						
	Weight						
	Reps						
	Weight						
	Reps						
	Weight						

Cardio

Exercise	Calories	Distance	Time

Water Intake _______________

Cooldown _______________

Feeling ☆ ☆ ☆ ☆ ☆

Notes

Today's Goal _______________ Ⓜ Ⓣ Ⓦ Ⓣ Ⓕ Ⓢ Ⓢ

Muscle Group Focus _______________ Weight_________ Date/Time_________

Stretch ◯   Warm-Up ____

Strength Training

Exercise		Set 1	Set 2	Set 3	Set 4	Set 5	Set 6
	Reps						
	Weight						
	Reps						
	Weight						
	Reps						
	Weight						
	Reps						
	Weight						
	Reps						
	Weight						
	Reps						
	Weight						
	Reps						
	Weight						
	Reps						
	Weight						
	Reps						
	Weight						

Cardio

Exercise	Calories	Distance	Time

Water Intake _______________

Cooldown _______________

Feeling ☆☆☆☆☆

Notes

Today's Goal _______________

(M) (T) (W) (T) (F) **S** **S**

Muscle Group Focus _______________ Weight_________ Date/Time_________

Stretch ◯   Warm-Up ________________________________

Strength Training

Exercise		Set 1	Set 2	Set 3	Set 4	Set 5	Set 6
	Reps						
	Weight						
	Reps						
	Weight						
	Reps						
	Weight						
	Reps						
	Weight						
	Reps						
	Weight						
	Reps						
	Weight						
	Reps						
	Weight						
	Reps						
	Weight						
	Reps						
	Weight						
	Reps						
	Weight						

Cardio

Exercise	Calories	Distance	Time

Water Intake _______________

Cooldown _______________

Feeling ☆ ☆ ☆ ☆ ☆

Notes

Today's Goal ___________________   (M) (T) (W) (T) (F) (S) (S)

Muscle Group Focus _______________ Weight_________   Date/Time _________

Stretch ◯   Warm-Up ______________________________________

Strength Training

Exercise		Set 1	Set 2	Set 3	Set 4	Set 5	Set 6
	Reps						
	Weight						
	Reps						
	Weight						
	Reps						
	Weight						
	Reps						
	Weight						
	Reps						
	Weight						
	Reps						
	Weight						
	Reps						
	Weight						
	Reps						
	Weight						
	Reps						
	Weight						
	Reps						
	Weight						

Cardio

Exercise	Calories	Distance	Time

Water Intake ___________________

Cooldown _______________

Feeling ☆ ☆ ☆ ☆ ☆

Notes

Today's Goal ________________

(M) (T) (W) (T) (F) (S) (S)

Muscle Group Focus _______________ Weight________ Date/Time_______

Stretch ◯   Warm-Up ______________________________________

Strength Training

Exercise		Set 1	Set 2	Set 3	Set 4	Set 5	Set 6
	Reps						
	Weight						
	Reps						
	Weight						
	Reps						
	Weight						
	Reps						
	Weight						
	Reps						
	Weight						
	Reps						
	Weight						
	Reps						
	Weight						
	Reps						
	Weight						
	Reps						
	Weight						
	Reps						
	Weight						

Cardio

Exercise	Calories	Distance	Time

Water Intake _______________

Cooldown _______________

Feeling ☆ ☆ ☆ ☆ ☆

Notes

Today's Goal ______________   (M) (T) (W) (T) (F) (S) (S)

Muscle Group Focus ______________ Weight________ Date/Time________

Stretch ◯   Warm-Up ________________________________

Strength Training

Exercise		Set 1	Set 2	Set 3	Set 4	Set 5	Set 6
	Reps						
	Weight						
	Reps						
	Weight						
	Reps						
	Weight						
	Reps						
	Weight						
	Reps						
	Weight						
	Reps						
	Weight						
	Reps						
	Weight						
	Reps						
	Weight						
	Reps						
	Weight						
	Reps						
	Weight						

Cardio

Exercise	Calories	Distance	Time

Water Intake ________________

Cooldown ________________

Feeling ☆ ☆ ☆ ☆ ☆

Notes

Today's Goal ____________

(M) (T) (W) (T) (F) (S) (S)

Muscle Group Focus ____________ Weight________ Date/Time________

Stretch ◯   Warm-Up ____________________________

Strength Training

Exercise		Set 1	Set 2	Set 3	Set 4	Set 5	Set 6
	Reps						
	Weight						
	Reps						
	Weight						
	Reps						
	Weight						
	Reps						
	Weight						
	Reps						
	Weight						
	Reps						
	Weight						
	Reps						
	Weight						
	Reps						
	Weight						
	Reps						
	Weight						
	Reps						
	Weight						

Cardio

Exercise	Calories	Distance	Time

Water Intake ____________

Cooldown ____________

Feeling ☆ ☆ ☆ ☆ ☆

Notes

Today's Goal __________________   Ⓜ Ⓣ Ⓦ Ⓣ Ⓕ ⬤S ⬤S

Muscle Group Focus ______________ Weight_________   Date/Time _________

Stretch ◯   Warm-Up ________________________________

Strength Training

Exercise		Set 1	Set 2	Set 3	Set 4	Set 5	Set 6
	Reps						
	Weight						
	Reps						
	Weight						
	Reps						
	Weight						
	Reps						
	Weight						
	Reps						
	Weight						
	Reps						
	Weight						
	Reps						
	Weight						
	Reps						
	Weight						
	Reps						
	Weight						

Cardio

Exercise	Calories	Distance	Time

Water Intake ________________

Cooldown ________________

Feeling ☆ ☆ ☆ ☆ ☆

Notes

Today's Goal ______________

(M) (T) (W) (T) (F) (S) (S)

Muscle Group Focus ______________ Weight________ Date/Time________

Stretch ○   Warm-Up ______________________________________

Strength Training

Exercise			Set 1	Set 2	Set 3	Set 4	Set 5	Set 6
		Reps						
		Weight						
		Reps						
		Weight						
		Reps						
		Weight						
		Reps						
		Weight						
		Reps						
		Weight						
		Reps						
		Weight						
		Reps						
		Weight						
		Reps						
		Weight						
		Reps						
		Weight						
		Reps						
		Weight						

Cardio

Exercise	Calories	Distance	Time

Water Intake ______________

Cooldown ______________

Feeling ☆ ☆ ☆ ☆ ☆

Notes

Today's Goal _______________   (M) (T) (W) (T) (F) (S) (S)

Muscle Group Focus _______________ Weight_________   Date/Time _________

Stretch ◯   Warm-Up _____________________________________

Strength Training

Exercise		Set 1	Set 2	Set 3	Set 4	Set 5	Set 6
	Reps						
	Weight						
	Reps						
	Weight						
	Reps						
	Weight						
	Reps						
	Weight						
	Reps						
	Weight						
	Reps						
	Weight						
	Reps						
	Weight						
	Reps						
	Weight						
	Reps						
	Weight						
	Reps						
	Weight						

Cardio

Exercise	Calories	Distance	Time

Water Intake _______________

Cooldown _______________

Feeling ☆ ☆ ☆ ☆ ☆

Notes

Today's Goal _________________   (M) (T) (W) (T) (F) (S) (S)

Muscle Group Focus _______________ Weight________ Date/Time________

Stretch ◯   Warm-Up ____

Strength Training

Exercise		Set 1	Set 2	Set 3	Set 4	Set 5	Set 6
	Reps						
	Weight						
	Reps						
	Weight						
	Reps						
	Weight						
	Reps						
	Weight						
	Reps						
	Weight						
	Reps						
	Weight						
	Reps						
	Weight						
	Reps						
	Weight						
	Reps						
	Weight						
	Reps						
	Weight						

Cardio

Exercise	Calories	Distance	Time

Water Intake _________________

Cooldown _________________

Feeling ☆ ☆ ☆ ☆ ☆

Notes

Today's Goal _______________   （M）（T）（W）（T）（F）（S）（S）

Muscle Group Focus _______________ Weight_________   Date/Time _________

Stretch ◯   Warm-Up ____

Strength Training

Exercise		Set 1	Set 2	Set 3	Set 4	Set 5	Set 6
	Reps						
	Weight						
	Reps						
	Weight						
	Reps						
	Weight						
	Reps						
	Weight						
	Reps						
	Weight						
	Reps						
	Weight						
	Reps						
	Weight						
	Reps						
	Weight						
	Reps						
	Weight						
	Reps						
	Weight						

Cardio

Exercise	Calories	Distance	Time

Water Intake _______________

Cooldown _______________

Feeling ☆ ☆ ☆ ☆ ☆

Notes

Today's Goal _________________ Ⓜ Ⓣ Ⓦ Ⓣ Ⓕ ⬤S ⬤S

Muscle Group Focus _______________ Weight_________ Date/Time_________

Stretch ◯   Warm-Up _________________________________

Strength Training

Exercise		Set 1	Set 2	Set 3	Set 4	Set 5	Set 6
	Reps						
	Weight						
	Reps						
	Weight						
	Reps						
	Weight						
	Reps						
	Weight						
	Reps						
	Weight						
	Reps						
	Weight						
	Reps						
	Weight						
	Reps						
	Weight						
	Reps						
	Weight						
	Reps						
	Weight						

Cardio

Exercise	Calories	Distance	Time

Water Intake _________________

Cooldown _________________

Feeling ☆ ☆ ☆ ☆ ☆

Notes

Today's Goal _______________ (M) (T) (W) (T) (F) (S) (S)

Muscle Group Focus _______________ Weight_________ Date/Time _________

Stretch ◯   Warm-Up ____

Strength Training

Exercise		Set 1	Set 2	Set 3	Set 4	Set 5	Set 6
	Reps						
	Weight						
	Reps						
	Weight						
	Reps						
	Weight						
	Reps						
	Weight						
	Reps						
	Weight						
	Reps						
	Weight						
	Reps						
	Weight						
	Reps						
	Weight						
	Reps						
	Weight						
	Reps						
	Weight						

Cardio

Exercise	Calories	Distance	Time

Water Intake _______________

Cooldown _______________

Feeling ☆ ☆ ☆ ☆ ☆

Notes

Today's Goal _______________

(M) (T) (W) (T) (F) **S** **S**

Muscle Group Focus _____________ Weight_______ Date/Time_______

Stretch ◯   Warm-Up _____________________________

Strength Training

Exercise		Set 1	Set 2	Set 3	Set 4	Set 5	Set 6
	Reps						
	Weight						
	Reps						
	Weight						
	Reps						
	Weight						
	Reps						
	Weight						
	Reps						
	Weight						
	Reps						
	Weight						
	Reps						
	Weight						
	Reps						
	Weight						
	Reps						
	Weight						
	Reps						
	Weight						

Cardio

Exercise	Calories	Distance	Time

Water Intake _______________

Cooldown _______________

Feeling ☆ ☆ ☆ ☆ ☆

Notes

Today's Goal _________________   (M) (T) (W) (T) (F) (S) (S)

Muscle Group Focus _________________Weight_________   Date/Time _________

Stretch ○   Warm-Up _______________________________________

Strength Training

Exercise		Set 1	Set 2	Set 3	Set 4	Set 5	Set 6
	Reps						
	Weight						
	Reps						
	Weight						
	Reps						
	Weight						
	Reps						
	Weight						
	Reps						
	Weight						
	Reps						
	Weight						
	Reps						
	Weight						
	Reps						
	Weight						
	Reps						
	Weight						
	Reps						
	Weight						

Cardio

Exercise	Calories	Distance	Time

Water Intake _______________

Cooldown _______________

Feeling ☆ ☆ ☆ ☆ ☆

Notes

Today's Goal _______________

(M) (T) (W) (T) (F) (S) (S)

Muscle Group Focus _______________ Weight_________ Date/Time _______

Stretch ◯   Warm-Up ____

Strength Training

Exercise		Set 1	Set 2	Set 3	Set 4	Set 5	Set 6
	Reps						
	Weight						
	Reps						
	Weight						
	Reps						
	Weight						
	Reps						
	Weight						
	Reps						
	Weight						
	Reps						
	Weight						
	Reps						
	Weight						
	Reps						
	Weight						
	Reps						
	Weight						
	Reps						
	Weight						

Cardio

Exercise	Calories	Distance	Time

Water Intake _______________

Cooldown _______________

Feeling ☆ ☆ ☆ ☆ ☆

Notes

Today's Goal ________________   (M) (T) (W) (T) (F) (S) (S)

Muscle Group Focus ______________Weight_________   Date/Time_________

Stretch ◯   Warm-Up __________________________________

Strength Training

Exercise		Set 1	Set 2	Set 3	Set 4	Set 5	Set 6
	Reps						
	Weight						
	Reps						
	Weight						
	Reps						
	Weight						
	Reps						
	Weight						
	Reps						
	Weight						
	Reps						
	Weight						
	Reps						
	Weight						
	Reps						
	Weight						
	Reps						
	Weight						
	Reps						
	Weight						

Cardio

Exercise	Calories	Distance	Time

Water Intake _________________

Cooldown ________________

Feeling ☆ ☆ ☆ ☆ ☆

Notes

Today's Goal ______________ Ⓜ Ⓣ Ⓦ Ⓣ Ⓕ ⬤S ⬤S

Muscle Group Focus ______________ Weight________ Date/Time________

Stretch ◯   Warm-Up ________________________________

Strength Training

Exercise		Set 1	Set 2	Set 3	Set 4	Set 5	Set 6
	Reps						
	Weight						
	Reps						
	Weight						
	Reps						
	Weight						
	Reps						
	Weight						
	Reps						
	Weight						
	Reps						
	Weight						
	Reps						
	Weight						
	Reps						
	Weight						
	Reps						
	Weight						
	Reps						
	Weight						

Cardio

Exercise	Calories	Distance	Time

Water Intake ________________

Cooldown ________________

Feeling ☆ ☆ ☆ ☆ ☆

Notes

Today's Goal _______________   Ⓜ Ⓣ Ⓦ Ⓣ Ⓕ ⬤ ⬤

Muscle Group Focus _______________ Weight_______ Date/Time_______

Stretch ◯   Warm-Up ________________________________

Strength Training

Exercise		Set 1	Set 2	Set 3	Set 4	Set 5	Set 6
	Reps						
	Weight						
	Reps						
	Weight						
	Reps						
	Weight						
	Reps						
	Weight						
	Reps						
	Weight						
	Reps						
	Weight						
	Reps						
	Weight						
	Reps						
	Weight						
	Reps						
	Weight						
	Reps						
	Weight						

Cardio

Exercise	Calories	Distance	Time

Water Intake ________________

Cooldown ________________

Feeling ☆ ☆ ☆ ☆ ☆

Notes

Today's Goal _______________   Ⓜ Ⓣ Ⓦ Ⓣ Ⓕ ⑤ ⑤

Muscle Group Focus _____________ Weight________ Date/Time________

Stretch ◯   Warm-Up ____

Strength Training

Exercise		Set 1	Set 2	Set 3	Set 4	Set 5	Set 6
	Reps						
	Weight						
	Reps						
	Weight						
	Reps						
	Weight						
	Reps						
	Weight						
	Reps						
	Weight						
	Reps						
	Weight						
	Reps						
	Weight						
	Reps						
	Weight						
	Reps						
	Weight						
	Reps						
	Weight						

Cardio

Exercise	Calories	Distance	Time

Water Intake _______________

Cooldown _______________

Feeling ☆ ☆ ☆ ☆ ☆

Notes

Today's Goal _______________

(M) (T) (W) (T) (F) (S) (S)

Muscle Group Focus _____________ Weight________ Date/Time ________

Stretch ◯   Warm-Up _________________________________

Strength Training

Exercise		Set 1	Set 2	Set 3	Set 4	Set 5	Set 6
	Reps						
	Weight						
	Reps						
	Weight						
	Reps						
	Weight						
	Reps						
	Weight						
	Reps						
	Weight						
	Reps						
	Weight						
	Reps						
	Weight						
	Reps						
	Weight						
	Reps						
	Weight						
	Reps						
	Weight						

Cardio

Exercise	Calories	Distance	Time

Water Intake ___________________

Cooldown ___________________

Feeling ☆ ☆ ☆ ☆ ☆

Notes

Today's Goal _______________

(M) (T) (W) (T) (F) (S) (S)

Muscle Group Focus _______________ Weight_________ Date/Time_________

Stretch ◯   Warm-Up _______________________________________

Strength Training

Exercise		Set 1	Set 2	Set 3	Set 4	Set 5	Set 6
	Reps						
	Weight						
	Reps						
	Weight						
	Reps						
	Weight						
	Reps						
	Weight						
	Reps						
	Weight						
	Reps						
	Weight						
	Reps						
	Weight						
	Reps						
	Weight						
	Reps						
	Weight						
	Reps						
	Weight						

Cardio

Exercise	Calories	Distance	Time

Water Intake _______________

Cooldown _______________

Feeling ☆ ☆ ☆ ☆ ☆

Notes

Today's Goal _______________ (M)(T)(W)(T)(F)(S)(S)

Muscle Group Focus _______________ Weight_________ Date/Time _________

Stretch ○   Warm-Up _________________________________

Strength Training

Exercise		Set 1	Set 2	Set 3	Set 4	Set 5	Set 6
	Reps						
	Weight						
	Reps						
	Weight						
	Reps						
	Weight						
	Reps						
	Weight						
	Reps						
	Weight						
	Reps						
	Weight						
	Reps						
	Weight						
	Reps						
	Weight						
	Reps						
	Weight						
	Reps						
	Weight						

Cardio

Exercise	Calories	Distance	Time

Water Intake _______________

Cooldown _______________

Feeling ☆ ☆ ☆ ☆ ☆

Notes

Today's Goal _______________

(M) (T) (W) (T) (F) (S) (S)

Muscle Group Focus _____________ Weight________ Date/Time_______

Stretch ◯   **Warm-Up** ___________________________________

Strength Training

Exercise		Set 1	Set 2	Set 3	Set 4	Set 5	Set 6
	Reps						
	Weight						
	Reps						
	Weight						
	Reps						
	Weight						
	Reps						
	Weight						
	Reps						
	Weight						
	Reps						
	Weight						
	Reps						
	Weight						
	Reps						
	Weight						
	Reps						
	Weight						
	Reps						
	Weight						

Cardio

Exercise	Calories	Distance	Time

Water Intake _______________

Cooldown _______________

Feeling ☆ ☆ ☆ ☆ ☆

Notes

Today's Goal _______________   (M) (T) (W) (T) (F) (S) (S)

Muscle Group Focus _______________ Weight_________   Date/Time _________

Stretch ○   Warm-Up ____

Strength Training

Exercise		Set 1	Set 2	Set 3	Set 4	Set 5	Set 6
	Reps						
	Weight						
	Reps						
	Weight						
	Reps						
	Weight						
	Reps						
	Weight						
	Reps						
	Weight						
	Reps						
	Weight						
	Reps						
	Weight						
	Reps						
	Weight						
	Reps						
	Weight						
	Reps						
	Weight						

Cardio

Exercise	Calories	Distance	Time

Water Intake _______________

Cooldown _______________

Feeling ☆ ☆ ☆ ☆ ☆

Notes

Today's Goal _________________   (M) (T) (W) (T) (F) (S) (S)

Muscle Group Focus ________________ Weight_________ Date/Time_________

Stretch ◯   Warm-Up ____

Strength Training

Exercise			Set 1	Set 2	Set 3	Set 4	Set 5	Set 6
		Reps						
		Weight						
		Reps						
		Weight						
		Reps						
		Weight						
		Reps						
		Weight						
		Reps						
		Weight						
		Reps						
		Weight						
		Reps						
		Weight						
		Reps						
		Weight						
		Reps						
		Weight						

Cardio

Exercise	Calories	Distance	Time

Water Intake _________________

Cooldown _________________

Feeling ☆ ☆ ☆ ☆ ☆

Notes

Today's Goal ______________   (M) (T) (W) (T) (F) (S) (S)

Muscle Group Focus ______________ Weight________ Date/Time________

Stretch ◯   Warm-Up ________________________________

Strength Training

Exercise		Set 1	Set 2	Set 3	Set 4	Set 5	Set 6
	Reps						
	Weight						
	Reps						
	Weight						
	Reps						
	Weight						
	Reps						
	Weight						
	Reps						
	Weight						
	Reps						
	Weight						
	Reps						
	Weight						
	Reps						
	Weight						
	Reps						
	Weight						
	Reps						
	Weight						

Cardio

Exercise	Calories	Distance	Time

Water Intake ________________

Cooldown ________________

Feeling ☆ ☆ ☆ ☆ ☆

Notes

Today's Goal _______________

(M) (T) (W) (T) (F) (S) (S)

Muscle Group Focus _______________ Weight_________ Date/Time________

Stretch ◯   Warm-Up ____

Strength Training

Exercise		Set 1	Set 2	Set 3	Set 4	Set 5	Set 6
	Reps						
	Weight						
	Reps						
	Weight						
	Reps						
	Weight						
	Reps						
	Weight						
	Reps						
	Weight						
	Reps						
	Weight						
	Reps						
	Weight						
	Reps						
	Weight						
	Reps						
	Weight						
	Reps						
	Weight						

Cardio

Exercise	Calories	Distance	Time

Water Intake _______________

Cooldown _______________

Feeling ☆ ☆ ☆ ☆ ☆

Notes

Today's Goal __________________   Ⓜ Ⓣ Ⓦ Ⓣ Ⓕ Ⓢ Ⓢ

Muscle Group Focus ______________ Weight________ Date/Time________

Stretch ◯   Warm-Up ____

Strength Training

Exercise		Set 1	Set 2	Set 3	Set 4	Set 5	Set 6
	Reps						
	Weight						
	Reps						
	Weight						
	Reps						
	Weight						
	Reps						
	Weight						
	Reps						
	Weight						
	Reps						
	Weight						
	Reps						
	Weight						
	Reps						
	Weight						
	Reps						
	Weight						
	Reps						
	Weight						

Cardio

Exercise	Calories	Distance	Time

Water Intake ________________

Cooldown ________________

Feeling ☆ ☆ ☆ ☆ ☆

Notes

Today's Goal _______________ Ⓜ Ⓣ Ⓦ Ⓣ Ⓕ ⬤S ⬤S

Muscle Group Focus _______________ Weight_________ Date/Time_______

Stretch ◯   Warm-Up ____

Strength Training

Exercise		Set 1	Set 2	Set 3	Set 4	Set 5	Set 6
	Reps						
	Weight						
	Reps						
	Weight						
	Reps						
	Weight						
	Reps						
	Weight						
	Reps						
	Weight						
	Reps						
	Weight						
	Reps						
	Weight						
	Reps						
	Weight						
	Reps						
	Weight						
	Reps						
	Weight						

Cardio

Exercise	Calories	Distance	Time

Water Intake _______________

Cooldown _______________

Feeling ☆ ☆ ☆ ☆ ☆

Notes

Today's Goal ________________   (M) (T) (W) (T) (F) (S) (S)

Muscle Group Focus _______________Weight________   Date/Time ________

Stretch ◯   Warm-Up ___________________________________

Strength Training

Exercise		Set 1	Set 2	Set 3	Set 4	Set 5	Set 6
	Reps						
	Weight						
	Reps						
	Weight						
	Reps						
	Weight						
	Reps						
	Weight						
	Reps						
	Weight						
	Reps						
	Weight						
	Reps						
	Weight						
	Reps						
	Weight						
	Reps						
	Weight						
	Reps						
	Weight						

Cardio

Exercise	Calories	Distance	Time

Water Intake _______________

Cooldown ______________

Feeling ☆ ☆ ☆ ☆ ☆

Notes

Today's Goal _______________   (M) (T) (W) (T) (F) (S) (S)

Muscle Group Focus _______________ Weight_________ Date/Time _________

Stretch ◯   Warm-Up ____

Strength Training

Exercise		Set 1	Set 2	Set 3	Set 4	Set 5	Set 6
	Reps						
	Weight						
	Reps						
	Weight						
	Reps						
	Weight						
	Reps						
	Weight						
	Reps						
	Weight						
	Reps						
	Weight						
	Reps						
	Weight						
	Reps						
	Weight						
	Reps						
	Weight						
	Reps						
	Weight						

Cardio

Exercise	Calories	Distance	Time

Water Intake _______________

Cooldown _______________

Feeling ☆ ☆ ☆ ☆ ☆

Notes

Today's Goal _____________   (M) (T) (W) (T) (F) (S) (S)

Muscle Group Focus _____________ Weight_________   Date/Time_________

Stretch ◯   Warm-Up _________________________________

Strength Training

Exercise		Set 1	Set 2	Set 3	Set 4	Set 5	Set 6
	Reps						
	Weight						
	Reps						
	Weight						
	Reps						
	Weight						
	Reps						
	Weight						
	Reps						
	Weight						
	Reps						
	Weight						
	Reps						
	Weight						
	Reps						
	Weight						
	Reps						
	Weight						
	Reps						
	Weight						

Cardio

Exercise	Calories	Distance	Time

Water Intake _____________

Cooldown _____________

Feeling ☆ ☆ ☆ ☆ ☆

Notes

Today's Goal _________________

Muscle Group Focus ________________ Weight__________ Date/Time__________

(M) (T) (W) (T) (F) (S) (S)

Stretch ○   Warm-Up ____

Strength Training

Exercise		Set 1	Set 2	Set 3	Set 4	Set 5	Set 6
	Reps						
	Weight						
	Reps						
	Weight						
	Reps						
	Weight						
	Reps						
	Weight						
	Reps						
	Weight						
	Reps						
	Weight						
	Reps						
	Weight						
	Reps						
	Weight						
	Reps						
	Weight						
	Reps						
	Weight						

Cardio

Exercise	Calories	Distance	Time

Water Intake ________________________

Cooldown ________________

Feeling ☆ ☆ ☆ ☆ ☆

Notes

Today's Goal ________________ (M)(T)(W)(T)(F)(S)(S)

Muscle Group Focus _______________ Weight________ Date/Time _________

Stretch ◯   Warm-Up ____________________________________

Strength Training

Exercise		Set 1	Set 2	Set 3	Set 4	Set 5	Set 6
	Reps						
	Weight						
	Reps						
	Weight						
	Reps						
	Weight						
	Reps						
	Weight						
	Reps						
	Weight						
	Reps						
	Weight						
	Reps						
	Weight						
	Reps						
	Weight						
	Reps						
	Weight						
	Reps						
	Weight						

Cardio

Exercise	Calories	Distance	Time

Water Intake ________________

Cooldown ______________

Feeling ☆ ☆ ☆ ☆ ☆

Notes

Today's Goal ___________________   (M) (T) (W) (T) (F) (S) (S)

Muscle Group Focus ________________ Weight__________ Date/Time__________

Stretch ◯   Warm-Up ______________________________________

Strength Training

Exercise		Set 1	Set 2	Set 3	Set 4	Set 5	Set 6
	Reps						
	Weight						
	Reps						
	Weight						
	Reps						
	Weight						
	Reps						
	Weight						
	Reps						
	Weight						
	Reps						
	Weight						
	Reps						
	Weight						
	Reps						
	Weight						
	Reps						
	Weight						
	Reps						
	Weight						

Cardio

Exercise	Calories	Distance	Time

Water Intake ________________

Cooldown ________________

Feeling ☆ ☆ ☆ ☆ ☆

Notes

Today's Goal ________________ Ⓜ Ⓣ Ⓦ Ⓣ Ⓕ Ⓢ Ⓢ

Muscle Group Focus ______________ Weight________ Date/Time________

Stretch ◯   Warm-Up ________________________________

Strength Training

Exercise		Set 1	Set 2	Set 3	Set 4	Set 5	Set 6
	Reps						
	Weight						
	Reps						
	Weight						
	Reps						
	Weight						
	Reps						
	Weight						
	Reps						
	Weight						
	Reps						
	Weight						
	Reps						
	Weight						
	Reps						
	Weight						
	Reps						
	Weight						
	Reps						
	Weight						

Cardio

Exercise	Calories	Distance	Time

Water Intake ________________

Cooldown ________________

Feeling ☆ ☆ ☆ ☆ ☆

Notes

Today's Goal _______________ Ⓜ Ⓣ Ⓦ Ⓣ Ⓕ ⬤S ⬤S

Muscle Group Focus _______________ Weight_________ Date/Time _________

Stretch ◯   Warm-Up ____

Strength Training

Exercise		Set 1	Set 2	Set 3	Set 4	Set 5	Set 6
	Reps						
	Weight						
	Reps						
	Weight						
	Reps						
	Weight						
	Reps						
	Weight						
	Reps						
	Weight						
	Reps						
	Weight						
	Reps						
	Weight						
	Reps						
	Weight						
	Reps						
	Weight						
	Reps						
	Weight						

Cardio

Exercise	Calories	Distance	Time

Water Intake _________________

Cooldown _________________

Feeling ☆ ☆ ☆ ☆ ☆

Notes

Today's Goal ________________ Ⓜ Ⓣ Ⓦ Ⓣ Ⓕ ⚫S ⚫S

Muscle Group Focus ______________Weight________ Date/Time________

Stretch ◯ Warm-Up ____

Strength Training

Exercise		Set 1	Set 2	Set 3	Set 4	Set 5	Set 6
	Reps						
	Weight						
	Reps						
	Weight						
	Reps						
	Weight						
	Reps						
	Weight						
	Reps						
	Weight						
	Reps						
	Weight						
	Reps						
	Weight						
	Reps						
	Weight						
	Reps						
	Weight						
	Reps						
	Weight						

Cardio

Exercise	Calories	Distance	Time

Water Intake ________________

Cooldown ________________

Feeling ☆ ☆ ☆ ☆ ☆

Notes

Today's Goal _______________

(M) (T) (W) (T) (F) (S) (S)

Muscle Group Focus _______________ Weight _________ Date/Time _________

Stretch ◯   Warm-Up _______________________________________

Strength Training

Exercise			Set 1	Set 2	Set 3	Set 4	Set 5	Set 6
		Reps						
		Weight						
		Reps						
		Weight						
		Reps						
		Weight						
		Reps						
		Weight						
		Reps						
		Weight						
		Reps						
		Weight						
		Reps						
		Weight						
		Reps						
		Weight						
		Reps						
		Weight						
		Reps						
		Weight						

Cardio

Exercise	Calories	Distance	Time

Water Intake _______________

Cooldown _______________

Feeling ☆ ☆ ☆ ☆ ☆

Notes

Today's Goal _______________ Ⓜ Ⓣ Ⓦ Ⓣ Ⓕ ⬤S ⬤S

Muscle Group Focus _______________ Weight_________ Date/Time_________

Stretch ◯   Warm-Up ____

Strength Training

Exercise			Set 1	Set 2	Set 3	Set 4	Set 5	Set 6
		Reps						
		Weight						
		Reps						
		Weight						
		Reps						
		Weight						
		Reps						
		Weight						
		Reps						
		Weight						
		Reps						
		Weight						
		Reps						
		Weight						
		Reps						
		Weight						
		Reps						
		Weight						
		Reps						
		Weight						

Cardio

Exercise	Calories	Distance	Time

Water Intake _______________

Cooldown _______________

Feeling ☆ ☆ ☆ ☆ ☆

Notes

Today's Goal _______________

M T W T F S S

Muscle Group Focus ____________ Weight_______ Date/Time_______

Stretch ◯   Warm-Up ______________________________

Strength Training

Exercise		Set 1	Set 2	Set 3	Set 4	Set 5	Set 6
	Reps						
	Weight						
	Reps						
	Weight						
	Reps						
	Weight						
	Reps						
	Weight						
	Reps						
	Weight						
	Reps						
	Weight						
	Reps						
	Weight						
	Reps						
	Weight						
	Reps						
	Weight						
	Reps						
	Weight						

Cardio

Exercise	Calories	Distance	Time

Water Intake _______________

Cooldown _______________

Feeling ☆ ☆ ☆ ☆ ☆

Notes

Today's Goal ________________   (M) (T) (W) (T) (F) (S) (S)

Muscle Group Focus _____________ Weight________ Date/Time________

Stretch ◯   Warm-Up _______________________________

Strength Training

Exercise		Set 1	Set 2	Set 3	Set 4	Set 5	Set 6
	Reps						
	Weight						
	Reps						
	Weight						
	Reps						
	Weight						
	Reps						
	Weight						
	Reps						
	Weight						
	Reps						
	Weight						
	Reps						
	Weight						
	Reps						
	Weight						
	Reps						
	Weight						
	Reps						
	Weight						

Cardio

Exercise	Calories	Distance	Time

Water Intake ______________

Cooldown _____________

Feeling ☆ ☆ ☆ ☆ ☆

Notes

Today's Goal _________________ (M) (T) (W) (T) (F) (S) (S)

Muscle Group Focus _________________ Weight_________ Date/Time_________

Stretch ◯   Warm-Up ____

Strength Training

Exercise		Set 1	Set 2	Set 3	Set 4	Set 5	Set 6
	Reps						
	Weight						
	Reps						
	Weight						
	Reps						
	Weight						
	Reps						
	Weight						
	Reps						
	Weight						
	Reps						
	Weight						
	Reps						
	Weight						
	Reps						
	Weight						
	Reps						
	Weight						
	Reps						
	Weight						

Cardio

Exercise	Calories	Distance	Time

Water Intake _________________

Cooldown _________________

Feeling ☆ ☆ ☆ ☆ ☆

Notes